Yin Yoga

How to Enhance Your Modern Yoga Practice
With Yin Yoga to Achieve an Optimal
Mind-Body Connection

Olivia Summers

Published in The USA by:

Success Life Publishing

125 Thomas Burke Dr.

Hillsborough, NC 27278

Copyright © 2015 by Olivia Summers

ISBN-10: 1533274827

Table of Contents

Introduction

Thank you so much for purchasing my book "Yin Yoga." My name is Olivia Summers and I'm a Certified Yoga Teacher and one of my many passions is the topic of Yin Yoga.

So many students that I'm introduced to have not even heard of the practice of yin yoga and for that reason, I've decided to write a book on one of my favorite forms of yoga.

The basis of the practice, however, does not stand alone. There could be no 'yin' without the 'yang.' Therefore it is fundamental that anyone wishing to practice yin yoga does so with the emotional, mental and physical intent to balance it with other "yang" forms of yoga such as hatha or ashtanga.

Why is this the case? Well, yin yoga is the calming and soothing—whereas yang yoga recharges and invigorates us. Obviously both types of yoga are needed, but in our modern world the emphasis is placed on yang activities, without much regard for our body's need for the yin side of things. This leaves us imbalanced and feeling off kilter.

Yin yoga has the ability to retrain our minds and bodies to become better at dealing with chaos and distraction—especially when you're having to hold certain poses for five minutes at a time.

By cultivating a quiet mind and outer calm through yin yoga, you'll be much better off when dealing with the stress that life throws your way. Not to mention your joints and tissues will be much better off because of it.

So if you're curious as to how to make yin yoga a part of your daily yoga practice, then keep reading!

The Evolution of Yin Yoga
How Did it Come to Be?

Relatively speaking, yin yoga is not a new development. The yin side of yoga has always been around. However, it wasn't until yoga teacher, Sarah Powers introduced her students to the idea of yin poses to counterbalance the more yang poses in their routine that the idea of "yin yoga" really took off in popularity.

Sarah had come to know yin yoga through the teachings of Paul Grilley—a Taoist Yoga practitioner from California and helped him spread the knowledge to the rest of the Western culture.

Hatha—the more "yang" style of yoga has been around in American culture since the early 1900's. However, when it was first introduced, it was taught as a system of gentle, static stretches and was actually more yin in practice—which is probably why most people thought it was pretty boring back then.

However, around the early 80's the hatha and ashtanga styles of yoga became much more yang. The classes were fast paced and exciting— think Vinyasa Flow or PowerFlow yoga. So as you can see, what was once considered a 'yin' form of exercise, wasn't any longer.

I think this is where the need for a specific type of yoga that catered to the softer side of stretching arose. This is why Yin Yoga was born—out of necessity to balance out our yoga practice and ultimately the rest of our lives.

What is Yin Yoga, Exactly?

The practice of yin yoga, as a whole, is similar to other forms of yoga in the sense that it does offer the same objectives and goals to stimulate and create growth within our minds, bodies and spirits.

However, yin yoga has the ability to heal us on a deeper level than hatha or ashtanga forms of yoga. How? Yin yoga focuses on our ligaments, joints, bones and connective tissues, whereas hatha yoga tends to focus on stretching merely our muscles.

Yin yoga is the perfect way to supplement your yoga practice—no matter your experience level. The reason for this is because it complements the more yang styles of yoga that lengthen and contract our muscles by targeting our connecting tissues in our lower spine, hips and pelvis.

Yin Vs. Restorative Yoga

Many people, at first glance, might think that yin yoga and restorative yoga are one in the same. However, the only similarities that they have are that they're both done on the floor and you can do them in cozy socks.

Aside from that, they couldn't be more different. The whole idea of restorative yoga is to coddle your body and help it ease out of any pain or discomfort you've experienced in the past or from injuries.

When you're in a restorative yoga class you're being guided to relax and basically take a nap for the duration of the class. Sure you might feel a good stretch here and there, but it's very laid back and gentle.

With yin yoga—it is *not* meant to be comfortable. The whole point is to invoke change in our bodies—from our joints to our tissues to our cells. For the duration of each pose (which can be up to 5 minutes or sometimes even longer) you'll be experiencing some amount of discomfort.

Each minute held in the poses will feel like an eternity and you may feel like you'll never be able to walk again. However, by holding these static stretches for intense periods of time, you are giving your body a chance to re-mold and re-formulate the way your joints and tissues connect to one another.

With yin yoga you are pushing your body past what it's used to and taking it to "optimal." Obviously, in order to do that, you have to put stress on the body to invoke change. Pay attention to your body and remember some amount of discomfort is to be expected but **if you experience true pain stop what you are doing and reassess.**

If you can't tell the difference between "discomfort" and "pain" I recommend finding an experienced instructor in your area.

When we've spent *years* of our lives sitting and being dormant for the most part, we put a major toll on our body and its natural range of motion.

The good news is, though, with yin yoga we can reverse the damage that we've done to our bodies and become better than we were before, even. It might feel a little intense at first, but I encourage you to give yin yoga at least 4 or 5 sessions before deciding whether or not you're going to keep practicing.

Yin Yoga Essentials

The foundations of Yin Yoga, believe it or not, are rooted in Taoist beliefs. According to personaltao.com, the definition of Taoism is as follows:

"*A simple way to start learning the definition of Taoism is to start within yourself. Here are three easy starting steps to learning Taoism:*

1. Don't concentrate on the definition of the Tao (this will come later naturally).

2. Understand what Taoism really is. Taoism is more than just a "philosophy" or a "religion". Taoism should be understood as being: A system of belief, attitudes and practices set towards the service and living to a person's own nature.

3. The path of understanding Taoism is simply accepting yourself. Live life and discover who you are. Your nature is ever changing and is always the same. Don't try to resolve the various contradictions in life,

instead learn acceptance of your nature."

The concept of yin and yang originate in Taoism and is often referred to as 'taijitu'—the yin and yang symbol has come to symbolize Taoism throughout the world. This is where the concept of yin and yang yoga comes from.

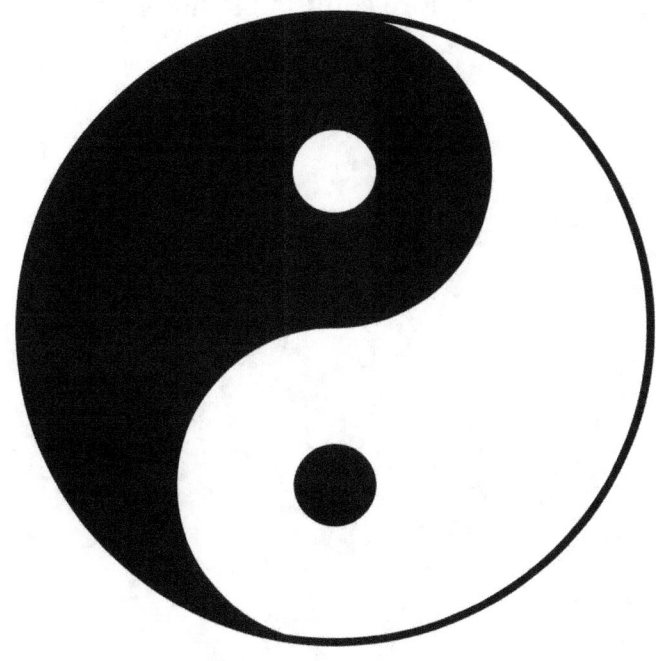

Taijitu Symbol

Differences in Yin & Yang

Yin and yang, by definition, are two halves that come together to make a whole. So in this sense, you can see why both yin and yang forms of yoga are required to balancing out your practice.

Translated, the word 'yin' means shady side and the word 'yang' is defined as sunny side. We see examples of yin and yang in our lives every day. The chart on the next page illustrates some of the more common forms of yin and yang.

Yin	Yang
Female	Male
Cold	Hot
Dark	Light
Inside	Outside
Slow	Fast
Downward	Upward
Dim	Bright
Moon	Sun
Earth	Heaven
Even	Odd

Plastic	Elastic
Water	Fire
Solid	Hollow
Mysterious	Obvious

As is evident in the chart, all aspects of our lives have a yin side and a yang side to them. Naturally, we must incorporate both of these aspects into our yoga practice as well. Otherwise, we're left with imbalance and chaos within our bodies. Even if we don't know it!

When we practice both yin and yang forms of yoga we learn how to serve our bodies in the best way possible. And it's not just all about the different types of poses either.

In yin yoga, *how* you practice is the biggest difference that you'll see and feel. When we practice the yin aspect of yoga we are nourishing, allowing and yielding—we become much more nurturing of our bodies.

At first, you might be a bit bored with this type of yoga practice and feel that it's not necessarily for you. However, I believe that if you give it a fair and open-minded chance, the way your body feels afterward will speak volumes to how much you truly need yin yoga in your life.

If you look back at the symbol for yin and yang (the Taijitu) you'll see that even within the darkness (or yin) there is a speck of light (yang)—and vice versa.

You can't have one without the other! Even while practicing more vinyasa flow type asanas you can spot yin qualities (i.e., breath control, mindfulness). So even if you weren't aware of it before this book, you have been practicing small portions of yin activities within your yang yoga practice.

So even though the concept of 'yin yoga' has been newly coined, it doesn't mean that it's a new way to practice, by any means.

However, the exercises in this book will take your yoga practice to a deeper level than you ever even knew was possible, but I bet your body (even if it was subconsciously), has been trying to tell you that there's more to the whole art of yoga than fast paced flow sequences that have become so popular in our Western culture.

Intuitively, though, I'm sure you knew there was more to it than that.

Physical, Mental & Energetic Benefits

So now that you know *what* yin yoga is...maybe it's time that I should explain *how* it can help you—physically, mentally and energetically. Keep reading to discover how yin yoga can improve all aspects of your life.

Physical Benefits

- Increase mobility of joints and hips
- Better lubrication and protection in joints
- More flexibility of connective tissues and joints
- Releases our fascia in our body
- TMJ and Migraine reduction
- Improves sitting ability
- Improves your other yoga practice
- Increases overall flexibility
- Better circulation throughout the body
- Balances internal organs

Mental Benefits

- Calms and balances the mind
- Lowers stress levels

- Deeper relaxation
- Helps coping with anxiety
- Increases clarity and focus
- Develops willpower
- Can help heal those with addictions, eating disorders or who have experienced trauma in their lives

Energetic Benefits

- Regulates energy in our bodies
- Increases stamina
- Helps increase our flow of prana throughout our body by stimulating meridian lines
- Balances your yang practice

As you can see, yin yoga provides many traditional and even more non-traditional improvements over your health than you would get by simply practicing ashtanga forms of yoga.

If you lead a balanced and healthy lifestyle by utilizing the yin and yang of your yoga practice, you will develop a well rounded and much more productive way of living. Not to mention you'll experience all of the amazing benefits that yin yoga has to offer.

Some Things to Keep in Mind

There are three important principles to keep in mind when you practice yin yoga. They're outlined below. Please read each carefully before proceeding to any of the poses.

Find Your Edge—When coming into each pose, do so slowly and deliberately. Speed is not your friend when it comes to getting into yin yoga poses. Even if you know that you "normally" should be able to go a certain depth into a pose, you should never start at the maximum. Take it easy to avoid injury.

Learn to Be Still—Yin Yoga is a very meditative way of practicing yoga and should be viewed as such. Is it going to be comfortable? Not in the slightest. But the idea is to quiet and "listen" to your mind and your thoughts as each fly by, learning to live in the moment without letting yourself readjust or find a place that's more "comfortable."

Hold it Here—The idea with yin yoga is to hold the majority of the poses for at least 3-5 minutes. By doing this we are able to retrain our joints and connective tissue to become more flexible and to lengthen and readjust themselves. Just face it:

you're not going to feel extremely comfortable here—that's not what it's about. Push through the discomfort and hold the poses to retrain your body.

With that out of the way, you're now ready to move on to the part you've probably been waiting for: the poses!

The Asanas

The following chapter outlines each of the different asanas in the yin yoga practice. You might notice that some of the poses are the same as the ones you'll find in regular ashtanga yoga practices, just with different names.

The name distinction is very important. Just because a yin pose might look similar to its ashtanga counterpart, does not mean that it's working your body in the same way.

Each yin pose will work much deeper into your connective tissues, ligaments joints, organs and even meridian lines of your body to promote an all-over healing effect on your body.

Pose 1: Anahatasana

Step 1: Start out on your hands and knees in tabletop position. Be sure to line your wrists up underneath both shoulders and both knees under each of your hips. Pull your shoulders inward and down the spine, then tuck all your toes under.

Step 2: Keep both legs where they are and then carefully walk both hands forward, allowing your chest to lower to the mat. In this position, tilt the pelvic bone back through the front of the legs. Keep walking your hands forward until your chest is about half an inch off the mat.

Step 3: Rest your forehead on the floor and press into your palms and into your toes.

Hold here for 3-5 minutes.
Do not do this pose if you have neck injuries or neck pain.

If you experience tingling in your hands or fingers, re-adjust or come out of the position, as this is a sign of nerve compression and we don't want to damage it permanently!

Adjustments:
- If you find you're uncomfortable, you can put a folded blanket underneath your knees to alleviate pressure
- You can also rest your chest on a bolster to keep the body relaxed

Joints Targeted:

Shoulder

Lower Spine

Upper Back

Meridians & Organs Targeted:

Urinary Bladder

Stomach

Spleen

Heart

Lung

Pose 2: Ankle Stretch

Step 1: Start by sitting back on your heels and place both hands behind you on the floor, making sure to keep your chest pressed forward.

Step 2: After a minute or so, bring both hands to the floor beside each leg, but again be conscious that you aren't leaning away from your knees. Keep the chest pressed forward and arch your back slightly.

Step 3: Lastly, hold onto both knees and carefully pull them in toward your chest, feeling a gentle stretch.

Try to hold here for 1 minute.

However, if there's a lot of discomfort then come out of the pose. If you feel sharp pain in your ankles or you have knee issues that make it uncomfortable then do not prolong the pose.

Joints Targeted:

Ankle

Meridians & Organs Targeted:

Stomach

Spleen

Liver

Gall bladder

Pose 3: Bananasana

Step 1: Start by lying on your mat on your back. Keep both legs together, straight out in front of you on the mat. Slowly reach both arms overhead and clasp at your hands or elbows.

Step 2: Now, with your butt planted firmly on the mat, move both your feet and upper part of your body to your right. Arch yourself to mimic the shape of a banana. However, be mindful not to roll or twist the hips up off the floor.

Step 3: Once your body feels comfortable here, pull your body even further to the right. If you're as far into the position as you can get, cross your ankles. Generally you'll want to place the outside ankle over the top of the inner ankle to feel the best stretch.

Hold for 3-5 minutes.

If you feel tingling in your hands, simply place a bolter under your arms or bring your hands down at your sides.

Also, be mindful of low back pain in this pose.

Joints Targeted:

Spine

Rib cage

Meridians & Organs Targeted:

Gall Bladder

Heart

Lung

Pose 4: Butterfly

Step 1: Start out by sitting on the floor. Bring both feet together and press the soles into each other.

Step 2: Slide your feet away from you, allowing the spine to round and fold forward.

Step 3: Your hands should be resting lightly on your feet or on your mat in front of you. Hang your head down toward your heels.

Hold for 3-5 minutes, but can be held for much longer periods if you desire.

If you have sciatica, you might not feel very comfortable in this pose.
If you feel any lower back pain, do not round your back—keep it straight.

Adjustments:

- If you're neck is stressed in this position you can support your head in your hands while resting your elbows on your thighs or a block.
- You can rest your chest on a bolster over your thighs to relax more.
- If your back hurts here, you can keep your legs in the butterfly position and simply lay back, flat on the floor.

Joints Targeted:

Hips

Lower Spine

Meridians & Organs Targeted:

Urinary Bladder

Gall Bladder

Kidneys

Liver

Pose 5: Half Butterfly

Step 1: Start out sitting on the floor. Bring one foot inward (in a half cross-legged position) while stretching your other leg straight out to your side.

Step 2: Now, fold forward and allow your spine to round out as you bring your torso forward between both legs.

Step 3: If you want an even deeper stretch, fold yourself forward over your straightened leg to stretch your hamstring more.

Hold here for 3-5 minutes.

- This is another pose that may aggravate sciatica, so practice with caution.
- If you have low back pain, avoid rounding the back.
- If you have sharp pains in your knees, engage the muscle in the top of your thigh or you can bring your legs closer to each other.
- Alternatively, you can put a folded towel or blanket under your bent knee for support or under the straight leg as well.

Joints Targeted:

Knees

Spine

Meridians & Organs Targeted:

Urinary Bladder

Liver & Kidneys

Pose 6: Camel

Step 1: Get on the floor with your knees hip width apart. Visualize yourself drawing your glutes up into your body, but keep your hips soft while you plant your shins and tops of the feet into the floor.

Step 2: Place your hands on your hips as you rest your palms on your butt with your fingers pointing down. As you inhale, keep your shoulder blades pressed back and your head high. Ideally you want to keep your thighs perpendicular to the floor, but if you're a beginner it's perfectly okay to give yourself some slack. If you can't go straight back to touch your feet you can turn slightly to one side and place your hand on your foot, then go back to the neutral position and place your other hand on your other foot.

Step 3: Make sure to lift your pelvic bone upward and focus on lengthening your spine and releasing pressure. As you do so place your hands against your heels and your fingers pointing down to your toes. Don't squeeze your shoulder blades together and don't tighten your neck or throat area.

Hold this pose for up to 3 minutes if it's comfortable for you.

Avoid this pose if you have back issues.

Adjustments:
- If you have neck pain, do not lay your head back—keep your chin tucked into your chest.
- If you feel less flexible, you can rest your hands on your heels or put a block between your feet for support.

Joints Targeted:

Spine

Shoulders

Ankles

Meridians & Organs Targeted:

Urinary Bladder

Kidneys

Spleen

Stomach

Heart

Lung

Thyroid

Pose 7: Cat Pulling Its Tail

There are two ways to get into this pose so choose which one would work best for you below.

Option 1
Step 1: Start sitting on the floor with both your legs straight out in front of you.

Step 2: Now, twist to your right and recline on the right elbow. Keep your right leg straight and bring the left leg forward to the side.

Step 3: Then, bend your right leg back toward your butt. Reach back with your left hand and grab the right foot, pulling it out and away from you.

Option 2
Step 1: Start by lying down in the floor. From this position, roll onto the right side of your body.

Step 2: Keep your right leg extended and then bring the left leg out to the side.

Step 3: Last, bend your right leg and bring your heel in to your butt. Reach back with your left hand and grab the right foot, pulling it out and away from you.

Hold this pose for up to 3 minutes.

Avoid this pose if you have low back issues.

Joints Targeted:

Sacrum

Lumbar

Rib Cage

Meridians & Organs Targeted:

Spleen

Stomach

Urinary Bladder

Kidneys

Gall Bladder

Pose 8: Caterpillar

Step 1: Start by sitting on a cushion or thick mat with both of your legs extended out in front of your body.

Step 2: Carefully and slowly fold your torso forward over your legs, letting your back round out.

Hold this pose for 3-5 minutes or longer if possible.

Avoid this pose if you have sciatica and feel that this aggravates it.

If you have low back pain keep your back straight.

Adjustments:

- If hamstrings are too tight, add a bolster underneath your knees to help with support.
- You can also add more cushions underneath your butt.
- If you need to you can also rest your head in your hands.
- This pose can also be performed in legs-up-the-wall fashion.
- If your knees feel strained, add a folded towel or blanket underneath for support.

Joints Targeted:

Spine

Meridians & Organs Targeted:

Urinary Bladder

Pose 9: Child's Pose

Step 1: Get into a kneeling position on the floor and sit back on your heels. Separate your knees hip width apart.

Step 2: As you exhale, lay your torso down on the mat between your thighs. Once you're settled in, lengthen the tailbone and neck.

Step 3: Now you can position your hands either straight out in front of you, palms toward the ground or you can place them at your sides palms facing up. Whatever is most comfortable to you. After all, this is a resting pose.

Hold this pose for 3-5 minutes, or however long feels comfortable to you.

Avoid this pose if you are pregnant, have diarrhea or you just ate a meal.

Adjustments:
- If you need to, feel free to place arms out in front of you.

- If you're not flexible enough to rest your butt on your heels, support your neck by placing the forehead on a bolster or on your hands.
- There's no need to keep the knees together. If it's more comfortable, separate them wider.
- You can also add a bolster under your chest for added support.

Joints Targeted:

Spine

Ankle

Meridians & Organs Targeted:

Spleen

Stomach

Kidneys

Urinary Bladder

Pose 10: Dangling

Step 1: Stand in Mountain pose with your hands on your hips. As you exhale, bend slowly forward at your hips. At the same time you should be drawing your stomach inward and engaging your abdominal muscles. You want to focus on lengthening your mid-section as you descend.

Step 2: Now, bend slightly at the knees and fold your body forward while clasping at your elbows with the opposite hands.

Step 3: Press your heels into the floor and lift your butt into the air. As you inhale, focus on lengthening your mid-section. As you exhale release yourself deeper into the forward bend and let your knees bend even more.

Step 4: Be mindful of your neck and keep it loose—let it hang freely.

Hold this pose for 2 minutes at a time, in multiple sessions since it's so intense.

Avoid this pose if you have high blood pressure, glaucoma or diabetes.

Adjustments:
- If you have back pain, bend the knees quite a bit to alleviate the pressure. Also, try resting the elbows on the thighs.
- If you have low back pain, keep the back straightened.

Joints Targeted:

Spine

Meridians & Organs Targeted:

Urinary Bladder

Liver

Spleen

Kidneys

Pose 11: Deer

Step 1: Start out by getting into the Butterfly pose on your mat. Then, swing the right leg back behind your body so that your foot is positioned behind your hip.

Step 2: Next, move your front leg away from you and attempt to make a right angle with your front knee.

Step 3: Move your back foot away from your hip until it feels like you're tipping forward and away from your foot, being mindful to keep your butt firmly on the mat.

Hold this pose for only up to 1 minute.

Avoid or be wary of this pose if you have knee problems. If you do try this pose, be sure to keep from rotating your hip.

Joints Targeted:
Hips

Meridians & Organs Targeted:

Gall Bladder

Liver

Kidneys

Stomach

Spleen

Pose 12: Dragons

Baby Dragon

Step 1: Start out in Downward Dog and then bring one foot forward between your hands.

Step 2: Walk your front foot forwards until your knee is positioned directly above your heel.

Step 3: Extend your back knee out behind you as far as you can, while keeping both hands on either side of your front foot.

Hold for 3-5 minutes.

Avoid if you have knee or ankle problems.

Adjustments:

- If you need to, you can put a folded towel or blanket under the back knee for extra support.
- You can also add a bolster or blanket under your shin or ankle if you need to.

Joints Targeted:

Hips

Ankles

Lower back

Meridians & Organs Targeted:

Stomach

Spleen

Liver

Gall Bladder

Kidneys

Alternative Variations:

Dragon Flying High

Rest your hands or arms on your front thigh and push chest out and forward. This will increase the weight over your hips.

Dragon Flying Low

Place both hands on the inside of your front foot and walk them forward as you lower your hips. If you want more of a stretch, rest your forearms on the floor or bolster or a block.

Twisted Dragon

Use one hand to push your front knee to the side, while the

other hand and forearm are pressed down into the mat as your chest is rotated and pushed up towards the ceiling.

Winged Dragon

Put both hands on the mat and push your right knee outward toward the mat in a gentle "flapping" sort of motion. Roll onto the outside edge of your foot and then hold here. You can also come down on your forearms or rest them on a bolster or block.

Overstepping Dragon

From the original Baby Dragon pose, move your front knee far forward and also slide the back heel out behind you until it's just slightly lifted off the mat.

Dragon Splits

Straighten both of your legs out into the splits position and support your front hip with a bolster positioned under your butt. You can either sit up tall or fold the torso forward for different stretches.

Fire-Breathing Dragon

Start out in Baby Dragon and then tuck your back toes under

as you lift your knee up off the mat. This will put extra weight on your hips and help to increase your stretch.

Pose 13: Frog

Step 1: Start out by getting into Child's Pose and then move both of your hands forward, extending them straight out in front of you.

Step 2: Keep your knees separate, but stay sitting on your heels.

Step 3: Lift your hips higher, until they're in line with your knees, but be sure to keep your feet together—this is known as Half Frog.

Step 4: Separate your feet as wide as your knees—this is Full Frog.

Hold in this pose for 3-5 minutes.

Avoid doing this pose if you have back pain, knee problems or are prone to get tingling in your hands.

<u>Adjustments:</u>

- If you have neck pain, rest your forehead on the floor instead of your chin or place it on a bolster.
- You can allow your hips to shift forward if there's too much pressure.

Joints Targeted:

Hips

Lower Back

Shoulders

Meridians & Organs Targeted:

Kidneys

Liver

Spleen

Heart

Lungs

Small & Large Intestines

Pose 14: Happy Baby

Step 1: Lie on the floor on your back. As you exhale, bring your knees into your stomach.

Step 2: On an inhale, grab the outside of both feet and open your knees up a little wider than the width of your torso. Pull your feet up towards your armpits.

Step 3: Bring both ankles directly over your knees, making your shins perpendicular to the floor as you flex through your heels. Gently push up with your feet while at the same time pulling your hands down to create a resistant stretch.

Hold here for up to 5 minutes.

Avoid if you are menstruating or if you have high blood pressure.

Adjustments:
- If you aren't flexible enough to grab your feet you can instead hold onto the backs of your thighs.

- Alternatively, you can use a belt or strap to hold your feet if you feel too tight or simply perform this pose against the wall—pushing into the wall with both feet.
- After a few minutes of engaging the stretch, just relax here in this position for several more minutes.

Joints Targeted:

Hips

Lumbar Spine

Meridians & Organs Targeted:

Kidneys

Liver

Urinary Bladder

Pose 15: Reclining Twist

Step 1: Start by lying on your back on the mat. Bring both knees up and into your chest, then open both arms out to your sides (like wings) and slowly lower your knees to one side.

Step 2: If you can't keep your shoulders flat on the floor, try placing a folded blanket or bolster underneath your bent knees.

Hold this pose for 3-5 minutes, playing around with the stretch and repeating on the opposite side for the same length of time.

Avoid this pose if you have rotator cuff injuries or other shoulder problems.

Adjustments:
- Raise or lower your knees to feel the stretch in different parts of your spine.
- If you want a deeper stretch, bring one knee up into your chest and hold it with your opposite hand so that it comes across your body.

Joints Targeted:

Shoulder

Upper Spine

Lumbar Spine

Meridians & Organs Targeted:

Urinary Bladder

Heart

Lung

Small Intestines

Stomach

Gall Bladder

Liver

Spleen

Pancreas

Pose 16: Saddle

Step 1: Start out by kneeling on your mat with both thighs parallel and making sure your knees are positioned hip width apart. As you exhale, lower yourself back toward the mat.

Step 2: To do this, place your hands behind you and then slowly and carefully lower yourself onto your elbows, placing your palms flat against your lower back.

Step 3: Finish reclining back onto the mat or with the help of a bolster or folded blanket. Rest your arms down at your sides, or if you feel like you're flexible enough, extend them back behind your head.

Hold here for up to 5 minutes if you feel up for it.

Avoid this pose if you have a bad back, knee pain, ankle pain or any sharp, burning sensations.

Adjustments:
- In this pose, straighten one leg out in front of you for Half Saddle.

- If you feel like you can't bend further than your elbows, rest here on a bolster.
- You can also put a block between your feet and butt to help lift your hips.
- If you're reclined all the way back, adjusting your head so that the top is resting on the floor will help open up your throat.

Joints Targeted:

Lower Spine

SI Joints

Ankles

Knees

Meridians & Organs Targeted:

Urinary Bladder

Kidneys

Stomach

Spleen

Heart

Lung

Pose 17: Shoelace

Step 1: Start by kneeling on your hands and knees, then put one knee behind the other one, siting back between your heels.

Step 2: Alternatively, you can start by sitting back on your heels and then sliding onto one butt cheek. From here you bring your outside foot up over the opposite leg and move it towards the outside hip.

Step 3: Finally, you can also begin this pose by sitting in a cross-legged position and then bring one foot under its opposite thigh and the other foot over the top and towards its opposite hip.

Step 4: The goal is to keep from sitting on your feet—move them as far forward as you can and keep your butt firm on the mat.

Hold this for 3-5 minutes on each side.

Avoid this pose if you have sciatica and feel it would be aggravated. Also, if you have low back pain either avoid this pose or keep the back straight and not rounded.

Adjustments:

- If your hips feel tight here, simply sit on a bolster.
- If you feel it's too hard on your knees, try straightening your bottom leg. If the top knee is what's hurting, put a blanket or bolster under it.
- If you need to support your head with your hands when you fold forward you can.

Joints Targeted:

Lower Spine

Hips

Meridians & Organs Targeted:

Kidneys

Gall Bladder

Liver

Urinary Bladder

Pose 18: Snail

Step 1: Start out by lying on your back on your mat. Then, lift both hips into the air as you support them with both hands.

Step 2: Slowly and carefully start to round your back and let both feet lower on either side of your head until they are close to the floor as you can get them. Be cautious of applying too much pressure on your neck—the majority of your weight should be distributed on your shoulders.

Hold this pose for 3-5 minutes.

Avoid if you have neck problems, high blood pressure, glaucoma, vertigo or a cold. Also avoid if you have eaten recently, are pregnant or you're menstruating.

Adjustments:
- For your arms, you can either keep them on your lower back with the palms flat (beginner) or if you can straighten your legs out behind you then you can place your arms flat on the

floor behind your back—even clasping your hands if you're flexible enough (advanced).

- If you want a deeper, more challenging stretch then you can bend your knees toward the floor as well.

Joints Targeted:

Spine

Meridians & Organs Targeted:

Internal organs

Urinary Bladder

Pose 19: Sphinx and Seal

Step 1: Start by lying on your stomach on your mat. Then, position your elbows so that they're slightly past your shoulders on the mat. If you have too much pain or pressure in your lower back here, you can simply move your elbows farther up on the mat, bringing your chest closer to the mat—this is the Sphinx position.

Step 2: To get into a Seal pose, simply straighten your arms and lock them.

For Sphinx, hold for 3-5 minutes.
For Seal, hold for 1-minute intervals, several times.

Avoid these poses if you have back problems, a headache or any sharp pains. Also, be careful if you're pregnant, not to press your stomach into the floor—you can use a bolster under your pelvis and your forearms if needed.

Adjustments:

- For Sphinx pose, you can put a cushion under your elbows to feel a deeper stretch.
- In Sphinx you can also put a bolster under your armpits to make the pose easier.
- To release some of the pressure in your lower back, you can spread your legs apart more.
- Alternatively, to deepen the sensations you can put your legs together.
- If you need to, you can put a bolster or blanket under your pelvis or thighs to offer more support.

Joints Targeted:

Lower Spine

Neck

Meridians & Organs Targeted:

Urinary Bladder

Kidneys

Stomach

Spleen

Adrenal Glands

Pose 20: Square

Step 1: To get into this pose, start by sitting on your mat, with your legs out in front of you.

Step 2: Cross your legs, moving both feet forward until the shins are parallel to the edge of the mat—"square" to it. The key to this pose is that you should feel the stretch in your outer hips—**not** the knees!

Hold this pose 3-5 minutes, per leg.

Avoid if you feel like there's too much pressure in your knees or hips. Also be careful if you have sciatica or low back pain (keep the spine straight).

Adjustments:
- To stretch your lower back, fold forward.
- For a deeper hip stretch, place your ankle over the opposite knee and then tuck the other ankle under the opposite knee.
- If you feel like there's too much pressure in your knees, you can put a folder blanket or towel under them for extra support.

- To get a different stretch, try sliding your knees closer to one another.

Joints Targeted:

Spine

Hips

Meridians & Organs Targeted:

Liver

Kidneys

Gall Bladder

Urinary Bladder

Pose 21: Squat

Step 1: Start out standing with your feet hip-width apart and then lower yourself into a squatting position.

Step 2: Your arms should be in front of your body, hands in prayer position, with your elbows pushing gently into your shins or knees.

Hold this pose for 2-3 minute intervals—alternating with other poses.

Avoid this pose if your hips are too tight or you have knee problems.

Adjustments:
- If you can't flatten your heels against the mat, widen your stance or place a blanket or bolster under your heels.
- On the same note, if your knees are not pointing forward in the same direction as your feet. If they aren't, spread your legs wider or put a bolster or blanket under the heels.
- To get a deeper stretch in your hips, widen your stance.

- To work your ankles more, move your feet closer together—even touching.

Joints Targeted:

Knees

Hips

Ankles

Meridians & Organs Targeted:

Liver

Kidneys

Urinary Bladder

Stomach

Spleen

Gall Bladder

Pose 22: Straddle

Step 1: Start out sitting on your mat, legs spread apart as far as you can get them.

Step 2: Then, fold your torso forward so that you're resting the weight of your body on your hands, with both arms locked in a straight position. You can also rest the elbows on a block.

Hold this pose for 3-10 minutes.

Avoid if you have sciatica, low back pain (or keep back straight) or any inner knee pain.

Adjustments:
- To raise your hips, sit on a bolster or cushion.
- Rest your elbows on a bolster or block.
- To feel a stretch in your spine and hamstrings, fold the torso over one leg, then alternate.
- If it feels like too tight of a stretch in your hamstrings, put a bolster under your thigh(s).

- If you feel like you're flexible enough, try folding yourself straight forward onto your stomach and keep your arms out to your sides.
- If you need to, you can even bend your knees so that you're feet are flat on the mat.
- Twist, by folding your body over one leg and then rotate your chest toward the ceiling.

Joints Targeted:

Knees

Lower Back

Hips

Meridians & Organs Targeted:

Urinary Bladder

Liver

Kidneys

Spleen

Gall Bladder

Pose 23: Swan and Sleeping Swan

Step 1: To get into Swan pose, start by getting into Downward Facing Dog, then slowly move the right knee between your hands, leaning to the right a little. As long as your knee feels okay in this position, flex your foot and move it further up on the mat. If you need to, you can bring your foot closer to your right hip.

Step 2: Now, center your weight in your body so that it's evenly distributed. From here, you can tuck your back toes under and also slide your back knee away from your body. Repeat this several times until your right butt cheek is as close to the floor as possible.

Step 3: If you're going to get into Sleeping Swan, simply bend your torso forward so that your stomach is flat against the mat and your arms are raised over your head, flat on the floor in front of you.

For Swan pose, hold for 1-3 minutes.
For Sleeping Swan, hold for an additional 1-3 minutes.
Avoid if you have knee pain or your hips feel too tight.

<u>Adjustments (for Swan Pose):</u>

- Keep your weight back in your hips when lowering yourself.
- Keep your hands flat on the floor, arms straight or lower yourself to your elbows.
- If you need to, place a bolster under your chest.

<u>Adjustments (for Sleeping Swan):</u>

- Keep your weight back in your hips when lowering yourself.
- Keep your hands flat on the floor, arms straight or lower yourself to your elbows.
- If you need to, place a bolster under your chest.

Joints Targeted:

Lower Back

Hips

Meridians & Organs Targeted:

Liver

Kidneys

Stomach

Spleen

Gall Bladder

Urinary Bladder

Pose 24: Toe Squat

Step 1: Start by sitting upright on your heels, feet together.

Step 2: Then, tuck the toes under—focusing on staying on the balls of the feet, not the tiptoes. If you need to, reach down and tuck your small toes underneath.

Hold this pose for 2-3 minutes.

Avoid if you feel strain in your knees. If you have tightness in your toe or ankle joints then stay in the pose for a lesser amount of time.

Adjustments:
- If you need a break at any point, sit up on your knees to get rid of some of the pressure on your toes. When you're ready, sit back on your heels again.
- If you're in pain at all, get out of the pose.
- If you're up for it, you can add some shoulder exercises to this pose—like Cow Face or Eagle arms.
- You can also put a folded towel or blanket under you knees or a cushion between the hips and heels.

Joints Targeted:

Ankles

Toes

Meridians & Organs Targeted:

All lower body Meridians

Spleen

Liver

Stomach

Gall Bladder

Pose 25: Savasana

Step 1: As you lay on your back, focus on lifting the pelvis and sliding the tailbone down to spread out your lower back. Don't arch the back unnaturally and lengthen your legs, resting them hip width apart. Let the feet and legs roll outwards to their natural resting position.

Step 2: Raise your arms and spread your shoulder blades so that they are away from your neck. Rest them at your sides at about a 45-degree angle with your palms up.

Step 3: Visualize and lengthen the neck by placing your chin closer to your chest. Inhale deeply and then exhale as you sink your body into the floor and become quiet and still. Visualize your entire body and it rests and feel your eyes relax and your mouth and face soften.

Hold this pose for anywhere from 10-30 minutes or more!

The idea for this pose is that you're paying attention to the prana flowing into the areas that you just worked through your practice. You should always end each practice with the Savasana.

Yin Yoga Flows

The following Yin Yoga flows should be enough to get you started for awhile. After enough practice you'll probably feel comfortable enough creating your own Yin Yoga flow sequences or you can always take a class for further instruction.

Yin Yoga Flow Sequences

Beginner's Flow 1—60-90 Minutes

1. Butterfly Pose
2. Dragonfly Pose—over right leg
3. Dragonfly Pose—over left leg
4. Dragonfly Pose—down the middle
5. Sphinx Pose
6. Child's Pose
7. Seal Pose
8. Child's Pose
9. Shoelace Pose—right leg forward
10. Shoelace Pose—left leg forward
11. Happy Baby Pose
12. Reclining Twist—right side
13. Reclining Twist—left side
14. Savasana

For a 60-minute session, hold each pose for 3 minutes. For a 90-minute session hold each pose for 5 minutes.

Please note: You should take a "break" between each pose for 30-60 seconds by stretching in whatever way feels good to you.

Beginner's Flow 2—90 Minutes

1. Frog Pose—2 minutes tadpole, 2 minutes full frog
2. Child's Pose—1 minute
3. Sphinx Pose
4. Child's Pose—1 minute
5. Shoelace Pose—right leg on top
6. Sleeping Swan Pose—right leg back
7. Shoelace Pose—left leg on top
8. Sleeping Swan Pose—left leg back
9. Caterpillar Pose
10. Dragon Poses—right leg forward

    2 minutes Baby Dragon

    2 minutes Overstepping Dragon
11. Downward Facing Dog Pose—1 minute
12. Child's Pose—1 minute
13. Dragon Poses—left leg forward

    2 minutes Baby Dragon

    2 minutes Overstepping Dragon
14. Downward Facing Dog—1 minute
15. Child's Pose—1 minute
16. Reclining Twist—right side, 2 minutes
17. Reclining Twist—left side, 2 minutes
18. Savasana

Hold each pose for 4 minutes, unless otherwise noted.

Please note: You should take a "break" between each pose for 30-60 seconds by stretching in whatever way feels good to you.

Beginner's Flow 3—90 Minutes

1. Butterfly Pose—1 minute
2. Swan Pose—right leg back, 1 minute
3. Sleeping Swan Pose—2 minutes
4. Butterfly Pose—1 minute
5. Swan Pose—left leg back, 1 minute
6. Sleeping Swan Pose—2 minutes
7. Butterfly Pose—1 minute
8. Straddle Pose—3 minutes
9. Butterfly Pose—1 minute
10. Sphinx/Seal Pose—3 minutes
11. Child's Pose—1 minute
12. Dragon Poses—right leg forward

    1 minute Baby Dragon

    1 minute Dragon Flying High

    1 minute Dragon Flying Low

13. Downward Facing Dog Pose—1 minute
14. Child's Pose—1 minute
15. Dragon Poses—left leg forward

    1 minute Baby Dragon

    1 minute Dragon Flying High

    1 minute Dragon Flying Low

16. Downward Facing Dog—1 minute

17. Child's Pose—1 minute, knees apart
18. Frog Pose—2 minutes tadpole, 2 minutes full frog
19. Child's Pose—1 minute, knees closer together
20. Anahatasana—3 minutes
21. Half Butterfly Pose—3 minutes, right leg out to the side
22. Sit with knees to the chest—1 minute
23. Half Butterfly Pose—3 minutes, left leg out to the side
24. Lie on back with knees to the chest—1 minute
25. Twisted Roots—right side, 2 minutes
26. Twisted Roots—left side, 2 minutes
27. Savasana

Hold each pose as noted.

Please note: You should take a "break" between each pose for about 15-25 seconds or however long you feel is necessary.

Spine Flow—90 Minutes

1. Dangling Pose—3 minutes
2. Squat Pose—3 minutes
3. Dangling Pose—2 minutes
4. Squat Pose—2 minutes
5. Straddle Pose—5 minutes, over right leg
6. Windshield Wipers—1 minute
7. Straddle Pose—5 minutes, over left leg
8. Windshield Wipers—1 minute
9. Straddle Pose—5 minutes, fold down the middle
10. Deer Pose—1 minute, right side
11. Deer Pose—1 minute, left side
12. Caterpillar Pose—5 minutes
13. Tabletop Pose—1 minute
14. Sphinx Pose—5 minutes
15. Child's Pose—1 minute
16. Seal Pose—5 minutes
17. Child's Pose—1 minute
18. Lie on back with knees to chest—1 minute
19. Cat Pulling Its Tail—1 minute, right
20. Cat Pulling Its Tail—1 minute, left
21. Hinge—2 minutes
22. Happy Baby Pose—2 minutes

23. Sit with knees to chest—1 minute

24. Snail Pose—3 minutes

25. Cat Pose—1 minute

26. Reclining Windshield Wipers—1 minute

27. Reclining Twist—2 minutes, right side

28. Reclining Twist—2 minutes, left side

29. Savasana

Hold each pose for amount of time noted. Set a timer for each if needed.

Kidney Flow—90 Minutes

1. Butterfly Pose—5 minutes
2. Windshield Wipers—1 minute
3. Straddle Pose—5 minutes, over right leg
4. Windshield Wipers—1 minute
5. Straddle Pose—5 minutes, over left leg
6. Windshield Wipers—1 minute
7. Straddle Pose—5 minutes, fold down the middle
8. Tabletop Pose—1 minute
9. Seal Pose—5 minutes
10. Child's Pose—1 minute
11. Dragon Poses—right leg forward

     1 minute Baby Dragon

     1 minute Overstepping Dragon

     1 minute Dragon Splits
12. Downward Facing Dog Pose—1 minute
13. Child's Pose—1 minute
14. Ankle Stretch Pose—1 minute
15. Dragon Poses—left leg forward

     1 minute Baby Dragon

     1 minute Overstepping Dragon

     1 minute Dragon Splits
16. Downward Facing Dog Pose—1 minute

17. Child's Pose—1 minute
18. Ankle Stretch Pose—1 minute
19. Caterpillar Pose—5 minutes
20. Lie on back with knees to chest—1 minute
21. Happy Baby Pose—2 minutes
22. Windshield Wipers (lying down)—1 minute, moving knees side to side
23. Reclining Twist—2 minutes, right side
24. Reclining Twist—2 minutes, left side
25. Savasana

Hold each pose for amount of time noted. Set a timer for each if needed.

Hips Flow—90 Minutes

1. Child's Pose—1 minute, knees apart
2. Frog Pose—2 minutes tadpole, 2 minutes full frog
3. Child's Pose—1 minute, knees together
4. Shoelace Pose—5 minutes, right knee on top
5. Swan Pose—1 minute, right leg back
6. Sleeping Swan Pose—4 minutes
7. Square Pose—5 minutes, right foot in front of left knee
8. Windshield Wipers—1 minute
9. Shoelace Pose—5 minutes, left knee on top
10. Swan Pose—1 minute, left leg back
11. Sleeping Swan Pose—4 minutes
12. Square Pose—5 minutes, left foot in front of right knee
13. Tabletop Pose—1 minute
14. Sphinx Pose—5 minutes
15. Child's Pose—1 minute
16. Saddle Pose—5 minutes
17. Child's Pose—1 minute
18. Dragon Poses—right leg forward

       1 minute Baby Dragon

       1 minute Dragon Flying High

       1 minute Dragon Flying Low

       1 minute Dragon Wing

19. Downward Facing Dog Pose—1 minute
20. Dragon Poses—left leg forward
    1 minute Baby Dragon
    1 minute Dragon Flying High
    1 minute Dragon Flying Low
    1 minute Dragon Wing
21. Downward Facing Dog—1 minute
22. Twisted Roots—2 minutes, right side
23. Twisted Roots—2 minutes, left side
24. Savasana

Hold each pose for amount of time noted. Set a timer for each if needed.

Yin/Yang Fusion Flow—90 Minutes (by Saul David Raye)

1. Virasana (Hero Pose)—3 minute meditation
2. Neck Circles—1 minute left, 1 minute right
3. Shoulder Circles—1 minute backwards, 1 minute forwards
4. Heart Tapping—1 minute, tapping up and down sternum with fingers
5. Sitting Side Bends (cross-legged)—1 minute right, 1 minute left
6. Sitting Back Bend—1 minute
7. Butterfly Pose—3 minutes
8. Stand in Uddiyana Bandha—empty the lungs, then draw your stomach in, up and under the ribs
9. Stand and perform Agni Sara—empty the lungs, then slowly pump the stomach in and out
10. Press "Reset"—turn your right hand into a fist, then stick out the thumb. Hold the right wrist with the left hand, gently pushing the right thumb into your belly button. Relax your stomach with each inhalation, pushing deeper. If it hurts, stop.
11. Arm Circles—1 minute backwards, 1 minute forwards
12. "Hah" Breath Drops—keep your legs wide apart and bend slightly at the knees. Raise your arms up and as you inhale

deeply, shout "Haaah!" while dropping your upper body and arms between your legs. Use the momentum to push you back up on the inhale. Repeat 5 times.

13. Squat Pose—2 minutes
14. Dangling Pose—2 minutes, knees bent
15. Squat Pose—2 minutes
16. Dangling Pose—2 minutes, legs straighter
17. Dragon Poses—right leg forward

      1 minute Baby Dragon

      1 minute Dragon Flying High

      1 minute Dragon Flying Low

      1 minute Dragon Wing

18. Downward Facing Dog Pose—1 minute
19. Dragon Poses—left leg forward

      1 minute Baby Dragon

      1 minute Dragon Flying High

      1 minute Dragon Flying Low

      1 minute Dragon Wing

20. Cat's Breath—1 minute
21. Squat Pose—1 minute
22. Dangling Pose—1 minute
23. Roll up from Rag Doll to Mountain Pose
24. Step your feet apart 3 ft., turning them outward—then squat, lowering your hips halfway to the mat with arms out to the side—1 minute
25. Use hands to pull thighs apart—1 minute

26. Side Fold—1 minute, over right leg

27. Side Fold—1 minute, over left leg

28. Wide Leg Squat—2 minutes

29. Frog Pose—3 minutes

30. Reclining Windshield Wipers—1 minute

31. Happy Baby Pose—2 minutes

32. Reclining Windshield Wipers—1 minute

33. Sitting—1 minute

34. Shoelace Pose—3 minutes, right side

35. Shoelace Pose—3 minutes, left side

36. Straighten both legs, bounces fast and hard against the floor—1 minute

37. Bend your knees and bounce your feet on the floor fast and hard—1 minute

38. Hamsa Breath—2 minutes

39. Savasana—up to 10 minutes

Hold each pose for amount of time noted. Set a timer for each if needed.

Tailoring Your Practice

Everyone is different when it comes to his or her own yoga practice. That's part of what makes yoga so unique and appealing—it can become what *you need* it to be. In the following chapter we'll discuss how to develop your own yin yoga routine.

Yoga Flow 101

So maybe you've gotten to the point where you're getting bored with the yin yoga flows that I've provided for you or maybe you feel like you've mastered each sequence, or maybe you're not quite ready to take a class at a studio. Whatever the reason—this chapter will help you out!

In this chapter we're going to go over how you can create and develop your own yin yoga workout sequence to cater to your personal likes and disliked—or even to help with a specific part of your body that you feel needs some focus.

How To Do It

Writing up your own yoga workout routine can be both

satisfying and also a little nerve-wracking. But nothing beats being able to customize your workout to fit any physical setbacks or personal goals.

A lot of people like to attend yin yoga classes for the simple reason that they don't know how to practice yin yoga any other way. Well, today I'm going to empower you to build your own routine and practice getting your yin on anywhere, anytime— no instructor needed.

Ready? Let's get started.

Step 1: Take out a piece of paper and a pen and write down all your favorite poses. You don't have to know the proper name or Sanskrit term for each pose—you can identify them in whatever way makes sense to you so that *you* know what the pose is and what benefits it offers. Your list might be very long or quite short. If it's on the short side and you want your routine to be a little longer, you might need to refer back to the poses I've included in this book or even do some research online.

Step 2: Next, sort each pose into more specific categories—such as resting poses, twists, hip openers, back exercises or even by which meridian or internal organ the pose is targeting.

To ensure that you have a balanced routine, you'll want to include poses from each of the categories. You can also create a routine that focuses on a specific area of the body, but you won't want to repeat only this routine because your body will become off-balance.

Please note: unlike other forms of exercise, you want your muscles to be cool and relaxed before practicing yin yoga, so no warm-up exercises are necessary.

Step 3: Note that you should start your workout with a meditative chant or breath technique. This should be done every single time because it's *that* important. With practice, though, you should be able to calm your breathing much faster than you will be able to in the beginning. Just be sure to find a quiet spot where you'll be able to focus on only your breathing for at least five minutes—or however long you feel you need to.

Step 4: One of the most important parts of creating your own workout routine is to decide if you want your workout to be more focused on—hips, back, all around wellness, yin-yang fusion, etc.

Whatever you decide, it's important that the poses you pick match up to your expectations. For instance, if you're going for focus on your hip joints then you'll want to choose appropriate poses to fit this need.

Step 5: This step is the most important step in my book and something you should take to heart. Too many times in my classes I see students fleeing from their mats when we get to this part of our yoga routine, which is unfortunate because it's incredibly beneficial and essential to our overall well-being.

What is it? Well, at the end of every single one of your yin (or yang) yoga workouts you should include Savasana—or Corpse Pose. Even if it's not specified in the workout!

The reason being, your body and mind need time to adjust to all that has just happened in the last hour or so—we don't want to rush right back to the hustle and bustle of our daily lives before we process and reflect on the journey we've just been on.

By lying on your mat, completely relaxed and at peace, breathing deeply at the end of each workout you'll be able to experience a rewarding calm that is worth the 5-10 minutes of delay.

Please keep in mind these 5 essential steps when planning out your own yin yoga routine. If you're at all unsure about what poses are able to be combined safely and effectively then it's best to practice under the supervision of a certified yin yoga teacher.

Conclusion

It is my hope that by taking the time to read this book, you now have a better understanding of the importance of a balanced yoga practice that includes both yin and yang styles of yoga.

Before reading this book you may have been unaware of the differences or that both types even existed. However, I hope that after reading my Yin Yoga guide that you can implement Yin Yoga into your personal yoga practice and realize the key importance of supplementing your routine with it.

It might not seem like you're doing much, since the majority of the poses are simply being held for longer periods of time without much movement. But by doing this you're stimulating many of your internal organs and meridian lines of your body, which will only help to improve your health and overall well-being. Over time, I'm sure you'll start to see how vital Yin Yoga is to a well-rounded and balanced yoga practice.

www.ingramcontent.com/pod-product-compliance
Lightning Source LLC
Chambersburg PA
CBHW071215280526
45787CB00002B/689